THE DBT SKILLS
WORKBOOK FOR TEENS

Understand Your Emotions and
Manage Anxiety, Anger,
and Other Negativity to Balance Your
Life For The Better

The Mentor Bucket

TABLE OF CONTENTS

INTRODUCTION

There is no denying it—life has given you countless reasons to feel scared, angry, sad, and frustrated. Sometimes, the feeling may seem okay. Other times, it feels as if your emotions have taken you over, and they spiral out of control as if they've got a mind of their own. To make things worse, the consuming emotions start interfering with your studies, causing you trouble when you try to make friends or preventing you from achieving your goals and enjoying your teen years.

If your teenage years seem stressful because you can't balance school and homework with your social and family life, you are likely walking through an array of emotions. Perhaps, you easily get frustrated and upset because someone in your school is spreading lies about you, or you feel very anxious because you are under some sort of pressure to outshine everyone else to secure your future. The truth is, you can't keep living like this. You can't keep struggling when you are supposed to be enjoying your teenage years and starting to follow those dreams you have.

Of course, there has to be a way to handle the roller coaster of emotions you are experiencing, and your reading this book shows that you've been seeking answers. Luckily, you are in the right place.

If you are ready to take charge of your emotions, achieve your goals, and be the best version of yourself, you can apply Dialectical Behavioral Therapy (DBT) skills. These can help you understand and manage your fluctuating emotions, improve your self-awareness, overcome impulsive behaviors, and effectively deal with relationship issues.

As a teen, you are naturally programmed to seek added information from outside your familial nucleus and to enjoy receiving attention from your peers. During these years, your learning ability has changed from concrete to abstract. You've experienced a change that involves identifying as a separate individual from your family or parents and facing an emotional separation from them. You see yourself as an individual with a sexual identity, and you now identify with your peers and have the drive to learn and explore the world. Additionally, your bio-sexual development is now slowly kicking into full gear; you are beginning to feel your emotions as much stronger than ever.

As a result, you may start struggling with managing and regulating your emotions, impulses, feelings, and relationships. When you struggle to manage these aspects, you may start experiencing additional issues such as anxiety, trauma, self-esteem, and poor grades, among other things.

These days, parents are more focused on teaching their children about hygiene, safety, and expected performance in school. They find themselves neglecting to teach physiological and emotional self-care. Teenagers are often not provided with enough guidance and information on how to handle their emotions, physical wellbeing, and relationships. However, in this fast-paced, ever-changing world, teenagers need to learn more about their emotions and how to be in control.

DBT is an evidence-based therapy that aims to teach individuals how to manage their emotions and thoughts and to build healthier relationships. Using DBT involves learning how to use its skills, including emotional regulation, mindfulness, interpersonal effectiveness, and distress tolerance.

The DBT-supported skills are important for all teens to learn, whether they've been diagnosed with a mental illness or need an effective way to manage their emotions, including anxiety, stress, anger, and sadness. DBT will increase your self-awareness and equip you with the tools to master managing your emotions and building healthier relationships.

For many years now, DBT has helped teenagers and adults struggle with frequent mood swings, angry outbursts, impulsive/disruptive behaviors, anxiety and depression, alcohol and drug abuse, suicidal behaviors, poor coping skills, family/peer conflict, and eating disorder behaviors.

While some people are better at managing their emotions than others, DBT can come through for those who seem to always find emotional balance impossible. DBT can avail you of the skills needed to handle your emotions and the feelings you experience while going through the difficult stage that takes you into adulthood. When your emotions are managed properly, you will have the interpersonal tools to build healthier relationships and effectively manage your behaviors and actions.

This book is for teenagers who intend to learn skills to help them manage their emotions as well as for parents who want to understand what their teens learn and how to help them.

For over twenty years now, DBT has become widely known and practiced by clinicians to help patients struggling to achieve mental wellness. It is a model of therapy that was first created to help chronically injurious behaviors and the suicidal population. As a result of this approach, DBT is now an effective method to cure a variety of mental health conditions.

I first learned about DBT when working as a clinician and helping the populace in battling persistent and severe mental illness. For every ten clients I talked to, seven were battling mental health conditions that included anxiety, depression, anger, trauma, suicide, and Post Traumatic Stress Disorder.

Fortunately, I had just received my DBT training and could attend to them and serve their needs. For many years now, after learning all about DBT, I've been helping people by utilizing DBT skills for teenagers especially.

I want this workbook to serve as a means of reaching a wider audience because I know many people are experiencing emotional challenges and want to set themselves free from the shackles of a roller coaster of emotions.

This workbook has been written in an easy format for your understanding. It is divided into six chapters, with worksheets and exercises you'll want to work engage with. The workbook extensively discusses what DBT is, how it can help you, and how to use DBT skills to overcome emotional issues such as anger, anxiety, trauma, and Post-Traumatic Stress Disorder (PTSD).

We'll start this book by explaining all you need to know about DBT and why you should pay attention to this form of therapy. This will serve as a foundational chapter, whereas other ideas will be built on as we progress with the workbook.

Are you ready to start this exciting journey with me?

I think I just got a resounding YES from you! Then let's get started!

CHAPTER 1: DBT AND HOW IT WORKS

DBT may sound strange to most people, or perhaps they've heard about it but don't know what it entails. Well, newsflash: I was once like you. When I first heard of DBT, I immediately assumed it was a complicated treatment and wasn't willing to give it a chance until much later. I hope that won't be the case for you. Regardless, I will be making sure I break it down for easier understanding.

First, I would like to answer the question, "What is dialectal?" If you've hurriedly picked up your phone to do a quick search, then I am sorry to let you know that Wikipedia and Google aren't that helpful in making you understand this word.

They've defined dialectal with bogus words, making it even harder to understand what it really means.

When I ask people what dialectal means, I often hear them say "dialogue," "discussion between two people," "something related to two things," and "the way people talk, like their dialect."

Psychologist and creator of DBT, Marsha Linehan, defines dialectal as an integration of two opposites. In other words, dialectal is when two opposing things are being true all at once. It is the existence of opposites, for which people are taught two opposite strategies (acceptance and change). This implies that they will have to make positive changes to manage their emotions and forge ahead.

If that's still confusing, let me give you an instance to gain a better idea of what dialectal means.

Say you have a sister you love dearly. However, she is always busy because she is working two full-time jobs at the moment. You have a question you need to ask her, and you've been trying to reach her for days now to get the answer. Either she doesn't pick up, or she picks up and abruptly tells you that she will call you back. This has been irking you. You care about her and think she is a nice person, but her being unavailable most times is something you don't like about her. Well, this is actually a dialectal situation.

There are two opposing facts about how you feel about your sister, and they are true at the same time.

This brings us to the term Dialectal Behavioral Therapy (DBT). What really is it? What does it entail?

What Is DBT?

DBT is a cognitive behavioral treatment. While Cognitive Behavioral Therapy (CBT) aims to identify and change your negative thinking patterns through positive behavioral changes, DBT provides you with new skills for managing your discomforting and painful emotions, while at the same time reducing the conflict you may be having in relationships. The main goal of DBT is to teach you to live in the moment and have healthier ways of coping with stress, regulating your emotions, and improving your relationships.

Originally, DBT was developed for treating chronically suicidal individuals diagnosed with Borderline Personality Disorder (BPD). Currently, it has gained the attention of the populace and is now the gold standard of psychological treatments for people with different mental health conditions.

DBT effectively treats people who have difficulty regulating their emotions or people showing self-destructive behaviors such as substance abuse and eating disorders. Also, it can be used to treat trauma and post-traumatic stress disorder (PTSD).

DBT equips you with new skills to manage your emotions. It focuses on providing you with therapeutic skills in four key areas. The first is mindfulness, which focuses on improving your ability to accept and be in the present. The second is distress tolerance, and this aims at increasing your tolerance for negative emotions instead of avoiding them.

The third is emotional regulation, which entails providing you with strategies needed to manage and change the intense emotions that are causing you distress. And the last is interpersonal effectiveness, which entails techniques that allow you to communicate more assertively, command self-respect, and improve your relationships. I will be explaining more about the skills of DBT shortly.

Conditions That DBT Treats

DBT has been endorsed by the American Psychiatric Association (APA) as an effective treatment in treating BPD. Teens who utilized DBT have been reported as seeing improvements such as less anger, improved social functioning, less likelihood of relapse, less severe suicidal behavior, and more confidence in handling emotions.

Studies have revealed DBT to be an effective therapy that helps teens suffering from anxiety, depression, and trauma. Your healthcare provider or therapist may suggest DBT be used on its own or in combination with medications.

Conditions that DBT effectively treats include:

Borderline Personality Disorder

DBT has its history with borderline personality disorder (BPD); this was the first condition it was used to treat. BPD is a condition affecting how one feels about themselves. Having intense emotions and unstable relationships with others are characteristics of BPD. According to research, DBT can be used to manage these symptoms (Chapman, 2006).

Suicidal Thoughts

Dr. Marsha Linehan first discovered the connection between suicidal thoughts and BPD. She realized that using DBT to treat people with BPD significantly reduced the risk of attempting suicide, a key marker for people with BPD.

This totally makes sense because people who have suicidal thoughts also find it hard to manage their intense emotions, tolerate their distress, and communicate with people. DBT can effectively address these symptoms and help individuals develop useful coping strategies.

Self-Harm

Deliberately harming yourself can happen on its own or be due to another mental health condition. Individuals who attempt to harm themselves do so as a way to escape a painful experience or difficult feelings.

With DBT, they can learn better ways to cope with these painful emotions, urges, and memories. With DBT, the individual will learn to accept these feelings as part of their experience, form a tolerance for distress, and better regulate their emotions.

Eating Disorders

While CBT is highly effective in helping people with eating disorders, it is not suitable for everyone. Research has suggested DBT as an alternate treatment that may be beneficial in some types of these cases.

People with eating disorders usually engage in unhealthy habits to escape, manage, and control their intense emotions. Since this is the case for many people, DBT can teach the individual other, healthier methods for coping with these emotions. This type of therapy works best for individuals with a binge eating disorder or bulimia nervosa and is not too helpful for individuals with anorexia nervosa.

Depression

DBT wasn't created to treat depression. However, due to its core premise, it has been found to be effective in treating the condition. The therapy emphasizes tolerance and validation, which are both in short supply for people with depression. People with depression normally feel worthless, which creates an overwhelming sense of sadness and invalidates almost all aspects of their lives.

With DBT, they will be equipped with coping mechanisms that allow them to address the negative aspects of their lives and break free from depression. This process may take time, but it's highly effective in the long term.

Benefits and Effectiveness

Many studies have suggested that DBT effectively treats borderline personality disorder, proving its benefits. The founder of this therapy conducted most of the studies herself and discovered these benefits.

DBT focuses on validating your experience and encouraging you to love and accept yourself while pushing for self-improvement. This approach to mental wellness is what gives you the skills you need for the following:

Improving Your Relationships

When dealing with any mental health condition, it's always beneficial to have a good support network. Many other therapies have failed to take this into consideration, and they expect you to do it alone. With DBT, there is an advocacy for understanding the role social relationship plays in overcoming the challenges that follow a mental illness.

When you create healthy relationships with trustworthy and respectful boundaries, you will experience improved health and general wellbeing in different ways.

Going Beyond Mental Illness

Even though the initial aim of DBT is to reduce the symptoms in people experiencing mental illness, it can go beyond that. The skills of DBT can now be applied to other areas of life as well.

For example, research has revealed that mindfulness is helpful in wellbeing and other aspects of life. With this skill, you can experience an improved aspect of your home, work, and play.

Improving Your Quality of Life

One of the main objectives of DBT is to improve one's quality of life. Sometimes, we aren't in control of what happens to us, and we can't foresee the future. Some people will experience mental health challenges as an everlasting part of their lives, and accepting this as a fact is important in moving forward.

DBT can help these individuals by improving the quality of their lives — encouraging them to make changes and go in the right direction while letting them know that it's okay to experience difficulties. People experiencing disruptive and intense emotions can have their quality of life severely impacted.

Managing Stress

The features of DBT support you in building the skills that will help you manage stress and stressors. Many people struggling with self-harm, suicide, and risky behavior engage in these because they are stressed and can't manage their mental illness in better ways. With DBT, patients will accept their stressors and manage them with positive coping mechanisms.

Controlling Destructive Thoughts or Actions

When using the skills of DBT, you will likely analyze your behavioral patterns and thoughts, take note of the destructive ones, and replace them with positive and healthy ones. If you find it difficult to regulate your emotions, learning to control and replace them is a significant part of living a healthier and happy life.

Improving Self-Perception

DBT encourages recognizing strengths and improving weaknesses. With a combined effort of positive support and self-improvement, you can counter the negative self-perception that usually accompanies a mental health condition.

Finally, as you focus on facts rather than your emotions or judgments, DBT will help you improve your ability to respond positively and productively without engaging in destructive thoughts, behaviors, and self-blame.

DBT Skills

DBT comprises four core skills that are called the modules. These skills help you cope with emotional distress positively and productively. According to Linehan, the four skills are the *"active ingredients"* of DBT.

Here is what the four skills entail:

Mindfulness

This skill is about having awareness and accepting what's happening in your present moment. With mindfulness, you can learn to notice and accept your feelings and thoughts without judgment.

Mindfulness is broken down into *"what"* skills and *"how"* skills when used in the context of DBT.

The *"what"* skills aim to teach you what you should focus on. They can be:

- Your present
- Your thoughts, emotions, and sensations
- Your awareness in the present
- The separation of your sensations and emotions from your thoughts

The *"how"* skills teach you to be more mindful through the following:

- Taking effective actions
- Balancing your emotions with rational thoughts
- Using mindfulness skills regularly
- Learning and tolerating aspects of yourself through radical acceptance
- Overcoming the things that are hindering mindfulness. For example, doubt, sleepiness, and restlessness

Emotion Regulation

You may feel like you can't escape your emotions, and this makes you feel helpless. But with a little help, it's possible to manage your emotions no matter how overwhelming they feel.

Emotion regulation skills can help you learn how to deal with the primary emotional reactions that tend to lead you toward distressing secondary reactions. For instance, a primary emotion of anger may lead to feelings of shame, guilt, worthlessness, and depression.

With emotion regulation skills, you can learn to:

- Reduce vulnerability
- Identify emotions
- Solve problems in helpful ways
- Increase emotions that have positive effects
- Overcome barriers to emotions that have positive effects
- Expose yourself to your emotions
- Become mindful of your emotions without judgment
- Not give in to emotional urges

Distress Tolerance

Even though mindfulness is very effective, it isn't always enough, especially when you are experiencing a crisis. This is where distress tolerance proves very helpful. With DBT skills, you can get through challenging times without using destructive coping mechanisms.

During a crisis, you may apply certain coping mechanisms to deal with the emotions that come with the crisis. For example, avoidance or self-isolation won't help you, even if they give temporary relief. Other coping mechanisms such as an angry outburst, self-harm, and substance abuse will cause harm instead.

With distress tolerance skills, you can:

- Soothe yourself by relaxing and using your sense of feeling at peace
- Distract yourself until you feel calm enough to deal with the emotion or situation
- Compare coping strategies by listing their advantages and disadvantages
- Devise means to improve the moment despite the difficulty

Interpersonal Effectiveness

When you feel intense emotions and rapid mood swings, it makes it difficult for you to relate with others. Knowing what you want and how you feel is an integral part of building helpful connections. With interpersonal effectiveness, you can become clearer about the effects of your feelings.

Interpersonal effectiveness combines social skills, listening skills, and assertiveness training to teach you how to change the situation while staying true to your values.

The skills include:

- Building respect for yourself (self-respect effectiveness)
- Learning the right way to ask for what you want and then taking the right steps to get it (objective effectiveness)
- Learning to walk through conflicts in relationships (interpersonal effectiveness)

DBT Techniques

DBT utilizes three main approaches to teach the core skills we just discussed. It is believed that the combination of these techniques is what makes DBT effective.

The techniques are:

Skills Training

The skills training group is similar to a group therapy session. These groups last for 24 weeks and meet once a week for two or three hours. Despite this, some DBT programs repeat the skills training to design them to last for a year.

In the skills group, you will learn and practice each skill and talk through scenarios with others in the group.

One-On-One Therapy

DBT usually requires one hour of one-on-one therapy every week. During these sessions, you get to talk with your therapist about your feelings, what you are dealing with, and what you are trying to manage. Your therapist will also use this time to build your skills and help you by navigating your challenges.

Phone Coaching

Phone coaching is also a technique some therapists use to provide extra support between your one-on-one appointments. If you often need extra support because you usually feel overwhelmed, phone coaching can be very helpful. Your therapist will guide you on how to use DBT skills to overcome your current challenges.

CHAPTER 2: UNDERSTANDING YOUR EMOTIONS

In the previous chapter, we discussed DBT and how it works. This chapter will take things a step further by discussing emotions and making intense emotions more bearable with different exercises. When your emotions are less intense, they become easier to manage; this helps get you off the emotional roller coaster when you find yourself on one.

Naming Your Emotions

The first step in understanding your emotions is naming them. How do you describe your emotional state? Do you normally use words such as "upset" or "bad" to describe how you feel? The truth is, these words are generic and don't faithfully describe your emotional state. When you say you are "upset," what does that mean? Does it mean you are sad? Angry? Or anxious? Being upset can mean any of these, so it's important to be specific about how you truly feel to enable you to know what to do about the emotion.

So, how do you name your emotion? Let's quickly look at the exercises below.

Exercise: Naming Emotions

Many words can be used to describe the eight basic emotions we have. However, each word comes with a slight difference in the "feel" or "flavor" of the emotion. It's better to have more words for the emotions you feel to help you describe your experience.

Below are eight primary emotions with a list of possible words that match them. Write the primary emotion that best matches the possible words listed in the space provided.

The Primary Emotions are Anger, Fear, Surprise, Interest, Joy, Sorrow, Disgust, and Shame.

The list of possible words:

Alarmed: . . . .

Nervous: ....

Hot-headed: ....

Depressed: ....

Ecstatic: ....

Up-tight: ....

Joyous: ....

Revolted: ....

Hot-headed: ....

Infuriated: ....

Sorrowful: ....

Miserable: ....

Annoyed: ....

Down in the dumps: ....

Livid: ....

Giddy: ....

Grossed-out: ....

In despair: ....

Afraid: ....

Restless: ....

Jubilant: ....

Exercise: Naming your emotions worksheet

A time I felt angry was when:

_____

_____

_____

_____

A time I felt nervous was when:

_____

_____

A time I felt afraid was when:

A time I felt depressed was when:

A time I felt joyous was when:

A time I felt confused was when:

A time I felt disappointed was when:

The Role of Emotions (Information, Communication, and Motivation)

After naming your emotions, what next? This section will discuss changing how you think about your emotions. This will be done by looking at their role or the function they serve.

You might not be aware of this, but emotions have essential functions and are needed even though they sometimes feel uncomfortable. While you might just want to toss them away, emotions are still needed and can't be tossed aside. This is why it's important to know their functions and learn to accept them.

According to the workings of DBT, there are three main reasons you experience emotions: information, communication, and motivation. Let's quickly discuss these reasons below.

Information

Your emotions are there to provide you with the information you need, though they can be modified to ensure they're more suited to your requirements. For example, the emotion "anger" can make you aware that something is wrong with a situation you see as unfair already or one you don't like for a certain reason. The emotions "shame" and "guilt" may arise to make you realize that you are engaging in something that's against your values and morals.

DBT has taught us that our emotions communicate with us by giving us emotional information before the brain can process the information received from our senses.

For example, you are walking home with your friends, and you decide to take the park route. You take the lead, and when you look ahead, you see something dark and shiny coiled up on the side of the path you are supposed to take. Immediately, fear kicks in to stop you from taking a step further and to keep you safe from what seems like a poisonous snake. This is done before your brain even has the chance to process the scene.

Have you ever been in a situation where your emotions fed you with information that made you see that you needed to act in a certain way, but they made things different than how you would have liked? Perhaps there was a time when your emotions gave you information that made you act in a certain way without even thinking about the rationale behind it?

It all borders on your emotions serving the function of providing you with information.

Motivation

Another function of your emotion is to motivate you to act. For example, it's natural to feel angry when you get bullied. As a result, you get motivated to take action against the bullying behavior by informing your teachers or the school authorities about the situation. You can also be motivated to participate in school campaigns to increase awareness of bullying and how to prevent it. Without the emotion "anger" to fuel your actions, there is every possibility that nothing will be done to improve the situation.

Another emotion that can motivate you is "fear." Immediately as your brain senses something that is a threat, you enter a fight or flight mode that triggers you to either run away from the situation or to stand and fight. Whatever your action may be, your emotion motivates you to act.

For example, you've just left your friend's place. You're walking home, and it's almost dark because you had to stay late to work on a group assignment together. You hear a strange noise, and immediately your fight-or-flight response kicks in. All your senses become heightened as you're trying to figure out what the strange noise is all about and whether it's a sign of danger. Your heart starts beating quickly, and your muscles tense. Then you see a strange man walking toward you, and I guess your next action will be to run back to your friend's house to ensure your safety. Your motivation for taking that action was triggered by fear, and that's what will get you to safety.

Communication

Another role your emotions play is in helping you communicate effectively with others. Your emotions are connected to specific body language and facial expressions, making it easy to identify them in you and in others. For example, people around you can easily guess how you feel based on your facial expression and body language. You don't need to tell them that you are sad when you have teary eyes or are sobbing. You also don't need to tell them that you are angry when your fist is clenched and your face is red. By looking at your expressions, they can guess how you feel and try to help you.

Can you remember any situation where your emotion served the role of communication for you? Maybe you felt sad, but even without your mentioning it, a friend tried talking to you to cheer you up. Or perhaps you wanted to scold your younger sibling for doing something wrong, but because of the emotion they expressed, you changed your mind and consoled them instead.

It's important to know that even though your emotions exist to serve a purpose, they aren't fool-proof and shouldn't be treated as authoritative. Feeling a certain way about something doesn't make it entirely true. You need to evaluate the situation and check for facts before assuming it to be true. For example, if a meal smells good, that doesn't mean it must taste good. First, before you can conclude, you need to engage your sense of taste to know if the food truly tastes good.

Your emotions are like the senses that provide your body with information. However, you need to be careful to avoid having them lead you astray. For example, seeing a stranger walking toward you and feeling threatened doesn't mean that person intends to hurt you. Because you saw a shiny black thing in your path doesn't mean it is a snake or something harmful. We'll be discussing how to reclaim your emotions in the next chapter; in the meantime, know that your emotions serve a purpose even if they don't always do it perfectly.

Exercise: Checking the Facts

When you experience some emotion, e.g., anger, it can be easy to place too much importance on the emotion and blow things out of proportion. In this Checking the Facts exercise, you can discover whether you are blowing things out of proportion and also reduce the intensity of the emotion you experience.

To check the facts, ask yourself the following questions:

What is the event that has triggered this emotion?

What assumptions or interpretations am I currently making out of the event?

Do my emotions and the level of their intensity correlate with the facts of the situation or my assumptions of the situation?

The Connection Between Emotion, Thought, and Behavior

Emotion is a full-system response that can make a situation confusing; there will be a lot going on simultaneously with emotions. While you are feeling a certain emotion, you are also thinking certain thoughts that are triggered by the emotion, and as a result, you engage in behaviors that relate to the emotions you feel. Because of what I just described, people usually confuse their emotions with behaviors and thoughts.

There is a connection between your emotions, thoughts, and behavior; hence, the confusion. Changing your thoughts will affect your emotions and behaviors; likewise, changing your behavior will affect your thoughts and emotions. This is because the three areas are interrelated. Most times, if you are asked how you feel, the description you give usually ends up being your thoughts instead. For example, what would your response be if asked how you felt after realizing that a stranger was walking toward you? Your answer can be, "I just wanted to run as fast as my legs could take me" or "I wanted to get out of there fast." These explanations are your thoughts, and the emotions connected with these thoughts might be "fear," "anxiety," or "distrust."

The full-system response of our emotions usually happens automatically and very quickly, so we don't pause to process what is really happening before we act. Let's think about it from a different angle. Don't you think acting without pausing to think clearly is one of the reasons our emotions get us into trouble? For this reason, it is important to learn how to separate emotions from behaviors and thoughts.

The naming of the emotions exercise you engaged in earlier will help you separate your emotions from your thoughts and behaviors. Right now, it's left for you to figure out what exactly you are feeling versus what you are thinking and how you are behaving.

Let's use our earlier examples to break this down and give you a clearer picture.

It's getting dark, and you are walking home from your friend's place alone. You suddenly hear a strange noise. Your experience might be something like this: Oh! What was that (your thought)? You look around, trying to assess the scenario (your behavior), and you notice that you don't recognize any familiar face. You start thinking, what if people are following me? What if I get attacked (your thoughts)? You start feeling anxious and scared (your emotions). If it is someone dangerous, would I be able to fight the person off? No one I know can help me (your thoughts). From this thinking, your fear increases (your emotion). Suddenly, you have the urge to run and escape whatever it is (your thought). You start considering what you should do (your thought). Immediately, you turn around and run back to your friend's house (your behavior).

Now, we will look at how the outcome of this scenario can change if one aspect of the experience is changed.

It's getting dark, and you are walking home from your friend's place alone. You suddenly hear a strange noise. Your initial thought might be: Oh! What was that (your thought)? You are looking around, trying to assess the scenario (your behavior), and suddenly you see people you don't recognize. You start wondering who they are because they don't look familiar (your thought). You are curious (your emotion) and continue to observe them (your thought). You notice two teenage girls standing in the corner of the park (your thought). You realize that they are looking at the street sign and their mobile phones; they may be lost (your thought). You start considering what you should do (your thought). Since it is getting dark, you are a bit concerned about the girls (your emotion). Then you approach them to ask if they are lost and need help finding the right way (your behavior).

We've just described two different outcomes based on the same beginning. Can you now notice that your behaviors and emotions can be influenced by changing your thoughts about the scenario?

Do you understand the connection now? If you don't, let's look at one more example to help you grasp it.

One afternoon, you return from school and inform your parents that you scored a "C" on your Mathematics test (your behavior). Even before telling them, you felt disappointed in yourself for having that score, and you are worried about how you will cope (your emotion). You're not sure if it will affect your chances of getting accepted in your preferred college (your thought). After informing your parents, they express the same concern, and you are upset with them immediately (your emotion), thinking they are always disappointed in you (your thought). You then yell at them and storm off to your room (your behavior).

Now, let's look at how the outcome of this scenario can change if one aspect of the experience is changed.

One afternoon, you return from school and inform your parents that you scored a "C" on your Mathematics test (your behavior). Even before telling them, you started feeling disappointed in yourself for having that score (your emotion), and you are worried about how you will cope (your emotion). You're not sure if it will affect your chances of getting accepted in your preferred college (your thought). After informing your parents, they express the same concern, and you are upset with them immediately (your emotion), thinking they are disappointed in you (your thought). You notice this thought, and instead of reacting rashly, you talk back to it. You realize they are disappointed in you because they notice you are disappointed in yourself (your thought). You then express your worry to your parents (your behavior). They give you some reassurance, which helps you change your thoughts and emotions about your Mathematics grade.

Now, don't just say that was quite easy. What I've given are just examples to demonstrate the idea of the connection between your emotions, behaviors, and thoughts. It definitely requires lots of practice to change your emotions, thoughts, and behavior. The first step is to understand why and how it is helpful to you when you do change them. Then you will start practicing the examples in this chapter. Before we come to the end of this section, quickly practice the PLEASE exercise below.

Exercise: PLEASE

The PLEASE exercise will help you acknowledge the connection between your brain and body. It becomes easier to manage your emotions when you know how to manage your body and health.

It entails remembering to:

- PL – Treat your **physical illness**
- E – **Eat** healthy meals
- A – **Avoid** mood-altering drugs
- S – **Sleep** well
- E – **Exercise**

These suggestions above should be followed to ensure your body is healthy and happy, making it easier for your mind to stay healthy and happy too.

PLEASE Worksheet

What do I need to do to ensure that my physical wellness doesn't affect my emotional wellness?

_____

_____

_____

_____

_____

What changes can I make to my diet to ensure I achieve emotional wellness?

_____

_____

_____

What are the three main motivations I can use to avoid mood-altering substances?

What sleep issues should I discuss with the doctor?

What activities can I engage in every day to ensure I get enough physical activity for the day?

CHAPTER 3: RECLAIMING CONTROL OF YOUR EMOTIONS

Your emotions play a significant role in how you react. When you are in tune with your emotions, you will have access to vital knowledge that helps you make your relationships a success, make effective decisions, enjoy better communication, and take good care of yourself. While your emotions play an important role in your life, they can also take a toll on your interpersonal relationships, emotional health, and your life in general. When this happens, you will start feeling that they are out of control.

According to a Tarzana therapist, Vicki Botnick, any positive or negative emotion can intensify and get to the point where it becomes difficult to

The DBT Skills Workbook for Teens

control. However, by pointing it in the right direction, you can take control of the reins, which we'll discuss in this chapter.

First, let's look at how the thought process works so we can better understand how to reclaim control of intense emotions.

The Three Thought Processes

According to DBT, there are three things you apply when you do any thinking: the reasoning self, the emotional self, and the wise self. If you are riding the emotional roller coaster, you will most likely think by using your emotional self. However, other thinking perspectives are equally important for you to access the different states that will improve how you manage your emotions.

The following section will discuss each way of thinking to help you practice knowing your state of mind.

Reasoning Self

In this state of thinking, you use your logical thinking and are straightforward with your thoughts. You only consider facts and do not judge with your emotions. There are usually no emotions in the reasoning state, and if there are, they are minimal and won't affect how you act. An example of the emotional reasoning self is when you choose a college because of the courses they offer, the school's reputation, and the likelihood of getting employed shortly after graduating from there. This is instead of considering things such as whether you like the location of the campus, how close it is to home if you want to be visiting home, or if you have friends that will be attending the college.

Another example of being in your reasoning self is when you do your homework, and you aren't so frustrated that you want to throw your books away. Or when you follow your parents' instructions on how to do the dishes because they went out and will be home late.

Even though many people ought to be familiar with the emotional self, some are on the emotional roller coaster because they often disregard their values and emotions, acting outside of their reasoning and experiencing the subsequent negative consequences. This means that if you ignore what your values and emotions are telling you, you are probably not acting in your best interest, which may trigger emotional pain such as frustration, anger, and sadness.

Emotional Self

The emotional self is the one you probably already know. When you think and act from your emotional self, your actions are controlled by your emotions. When you feel angry, you tend to lash out at someone even if the reason for your anger has nothing to do with the person. Perhaps you feel anxious and want to avoid what's causing you anxiety. For example, you would rather stay at home and miss classes because you don't want to be part of the presentation scheduled to be held today.

By acting from your emotional self, you react from your emotions instead of choosing how you act. It will feel like your emotions are in control of you while you are just along for the ride. When in an emotional state, you're likely to do things you will regret later by acting impulsively in ways that usually come with negative consequences over time. For example, breaking up with your boy-friend/girlfriend because you got angry with them, skipping classes even when you need to get good grades, or getting drunk at a party when you are supposed to be preparing for your exams. These scenarios should sound familiar to you if you've been on an emotional roller coaster. Thankfully, it isn't static; there are things you can do to change your thinking style.

Wise Self

Engaging the wise self is when you balance your reasoning self and your emotional self. This is in between the two; you aren't choosing one or the other. With your wise self, you will consider both your reasoning and emotions while factoring in a third element—your intuition. When in a situation where your feelings creep in, you allow yourself to feel them and consider what your logic is saying about that. Then you listen to the little voice inside you weighing both the positives and negatives of the situation, which will eventually tell you what will be effective in the long term.

Can you recall a moment in your life when your wise self was screaming for your attention? Even when you don't listen to it, know it is somewhere inside you. It is important to know that what your inner wisdom signals you to do may not be easy, and it won't be what you want to do. However, it is what's best for the situation, for you, and for others around you.

Getting a Wise Self

Like with learning anything new, accessing your wise self may take lots of energy, time, and practice, especially if you are used to listening to your emotional or reasoning self. However, don't let this discourage you from trying. Like I mentioned earlier, even though it may prove difficult, it is accessible; at the end of the day, attaining the skill will be worth the effort you've invested in it. It is a skill that will bring calm and peace to your life, and this will help you survive the emotional roller coaster you will experience. As you continue practicing the skill, it will become more natural.

It is time to engage in exercises that will get you to your wise self!

Exercise: Opposite Action

The opposite action is a technique you can use to stop highly charged emotions and make them less intense. Your emotional responses are usually followed by specific behaviors, such as withdrawing from people after feeling sad, or engaging in intense arguments after getting angry.

We often assume that the connection starts from the emotion and ends in the behavior, not the other way around. The truth is, it is possible to invoke a certain emotion if you engage in behavior associated with that emotion. The logic here is that instead of engaging in what you normally do when you feel a certain way, why not do the opposite action? For example, if you feel sad, why not insert yourself into the midst of your friends and chat with them instead of withdrawing from them? When you get angry, why not talk quietly instead of yelling?

For guilt or shame:

When you feel guilty or ashamed, instead of withdrawing and avoiding the situation, why not repair the transgression by apologizing telling the person you've offended that you are sorry, making things better (doing something nice for the person), accepting the consequences of your action, ensuring you avoid making that mistake, moving on, and letting go of the emotions you feel?

For fear:

Rather than giving in and showing that you are scared, why not do the thing you are afraid of instead? Engage in activities and tasks, or go to events and places, that normally make you uncomfortable. Talk to people you are usually afraid of. Do things that will give you a sense of control and mastery over the situation. When you feel overwhelmed, break the tasks into smaller, more manageable steps.

For anger:

Rather than attacking the person you are angry with, avoid them and avoid thinking about them. Do not dwell on them, be nice to them rather than mean, and imagine showing them empathy and sympathy instead of blaming them.

For depression and sadness:

Don't avoid; be active! Engage in things that will make you feel confident and competent.

Opposite Action Worksheet

In the worksheet below, aim to follow the instructions written under the step section, which signifies what you should do. For example, under "Identify the feeling," your identified feeling can be anger as a result of feeling cheated, anxiety about spending time with others, or sadness when you are not listened to.

Then, as suggested in the examples above, do the opposite action of what comes to mind. When you feel anxious about spending time with others and you want to avoid them, face your fears instead by spending time with them. When you feel scared of doing certain tasks, get used to your fears by doing those tasks rather than avoiding them.

Step: Identify the feeling

Example: Anxiety about spending time with people and making friends

Your Turn:

For Example: I will make new friends and spend time with people rather than avoid them.

Step: Identify the resulting action

Example: You would rather be alone and bury yourself in work, convincing yourself that you don't have the time to make friends.

Your Turn:

Step: Do the opposite action

Example: Push yourself to mingle with people and attend gatherings.

Your Turn:

_____

_____

_____

_____

Step: Feel the opposite feeling

Example: Excitement about making new friends Relief because there won't be a "push-and-pull" about whether making friends is a good idea or not

Your Turn:

_____

_____

_____

_____

Exercise: Increasing Self-Awareness

The first area you should work on when making any change is your self-awareness. You need to be aware of your thinking style, and once you have an awareness of this, you can choose what to do about it. So, how can you have this awareness? *By Observing, Noticing,* and *Acknowledging.*

To do this, you don't need to write down what you observe and notice, but if you *can* write it down, that could be helpful. The idea is to bring awareness to your experiences as much as possible. Ask yourself, *What thinking style am I using at the moment? Am I really listening to my wise self? What is my wise self-telling me to do right now?* Do this repeatedly throughout the day. Notice what is happening inside you when you question yourself without any judgment and are just being mindful of the experience.

Self-Reflection Worksheet

It's important that you reflect on yourself when practicing healthy and productive behaviors. This way, you can know what you do well and the areas that need to be worked on. The following worksheet should be used to track your progress in encouraging healthier behaviors.

The situation that triggered the behavior

Are you happy with the behavior?

If you are not happy, what could you have done better? If you are happy, what's the positive result of the behavior?

_____

_____

What areas will you be mindful of to improve your behavior next time?

_____

_____

_____

_____

Exercise: Monitor your inner voice

Do you know that the words you use every day significantly impact your relationship with yourself and other people and things? Talking to yourself is one of the most natural yet underestimated skills you possess. It helps by increasing your motivation, stimulating self-reflection, and connecting you to your emotions. According to a study by Canadian professor Alain Morin, there is a pronounced connection between talking to oneself frequently and having a strong sense of self-awareness.

The quality of your inner speech is important; therefore, the more positive words you use, the better your sense of awareness becomes. Pay attention to your inner voice and how you respond to your failures and successes. The feedback loops your inner voice creates can be turned into a positive or negative experience, and since the way you talk to yourself is how you get to love yourself, it is crucial to be careful with your words.

Also, limit using words such as *"I can't,"* as that can create a negative attitude and limit your potential. It makes you doubt your potential or see a task as a burden.

Validating Your Emotions

Validating your emotions simply means being non-judgmental with your emotions. It entails accepting whatever emotion you experience. You don't need to like it, just be non-judgmental about having it and toward the emotion itself.

When you validate your emotions, you prevent the emotion from escalating and the control from getting away from you. This doesn't mean you are getting rid of the emotion—DBT's goal is against this. However, the aim is to reduce the intensity of your emotion to enable you to manage your emotions.

A very effective way to validate your emotions is by being aware of your judgment toward them. This is where the practice of mindfulness comes in, and we will be discussing more on that in the next chapter.

For now, let's focus on how you can stop judgments and accept your emotional experience in the following three ways:

Allow your emotions

Allow your emotions because by doing that, you are giving yourself permission to feel everything about the feeling you have. Instead of saying, "*I feel scared,*" the self-talk will be "*It's okay to feel scared.*" I need to make this clear—I am not encouraging you to like the feeling and I'm not saying that you shouldn't make an effort to change the feeling. You need to acknowledge that you have normal human emotions, and it is okay for people to feel that way. It doesn't mean you are a bad person, and neither is it the end of the world.

Acknowledge your emotions

The next technique is to acknowledge the experience. By naming or labeling your emotion, you validate it without judging it. This may seem basic or simple, but it is very effective.

Understand your emotions

You can validate your emotion by being aware of the emotional context. When you understand why you feel the way you feel in a certain moment, your emotion makes more sense. You may not always know where your emotions come from. However, remember not to judge yourself for whatever you feel.

The following mindfulness exercise will help change your attitude toward your emotions and yourself so you will validate your emotions in the long run.

Exercise: Loving-Kindness Meditation

The Loving Kindness Meditation (LKM) was formerly known as Metta Bhavana in the Pali language. Metta means kindness, love, and friendliness, while Bhavana means the act of cultivating.

This simple mindfulness practice is done in five stages and should last for approximately five minutes.

Here is how to do it:

Stage 1: Feel the Metta (love) you have for yourself by being aware; focusing on peace, calm, and tranquility. Say out loud, *"May I be happy and at peace,"* and *"May I do well and be fulfilled."* Repeat these to stimulate the Metta in you.

Stage 2: Think of a good friend of yours. Remember their good qualities, feel the affinity you have for them (the connection you have with them) and encourage the feelings to increase by saying, *"May they be happy,"* and *"May they be at peace."* Picture an image of a shining light (halo) moving from your heart to theirs.

Stage 3: Think of someone you know but feel indifferent about. You neither like nor hate them, but you feel neutral toward them. Reflect on their humanity and add them to your feelings of Metta.

Stage 4: Think of someone you dislike or hate—perhaps a personal enemy. As you think of them, avoid getting caught up in the feelings of having hatred for them. Instead, think of them in a positive light and send them Metta.

Stage 5: Think of all four people altogether — yourself, your friend, the person you feel indifferent about, and the person you don't like. Start extending the feeling to everyone around you, your neighborhood, city, state, country, and all of the world. Slowly relax and bring the meditation to an end.

By doing this loving-kindness meditation, you are developing a positive wave that spreads to everyone and everywhere from your heart.

Explain how you felt when you connected with your body and focused on your breathing? Write down the feelings you had.

What distractions popped in during the exercise? Any common themes with your thoughts?

Who did you recall that made you happy and have deep feelings for?

What feelings did you notice in your body when thinking about the person?

Who came to your mind when thinking of someone you didn't like? How does thinking about them make you feel?

What sensations and feelings did you notice after thinking of this person in a positive light?

What sensations and feelings did you notice when extending love to everyone?

Maintaining Emotional Balance

This is a way of maintaining balance in your life. You don't want to remain in your reasoning self, and you don't want to remain in your emotional self, although both states are helpful and needed sometimes. For example, your emotional self-comprises pleasurable emotions such as joy, love, and excitement, so you wouldn't want to miss out on these emotions even when they are intense. Also, you will need your reasoning self to help you think logically about things. In all of this, the goal is to access your wisdom as much as needed, balance your emotions with your reasoning, and use your intuition to make healthier and wiser decisions.

This should be something we do daily, not just when we have life-changing decisions to make. It could be something as simple as the decision you make to go to school early to have enough time to prepare for your exams.

There are times when you act out of your wise self, but you don't get to notice it. It's time you start really seeing it so that you can appreciate yourself when you use it. Note, it is equally important that you are aware when you're acting from your reasoning or emotional self because when you are in this state and aware that you are, you will have the option to move to your wise self.

Lifestyle Changes for Emotional Balance

For many years now, research has revealed the connection between the mind and the body, knowing that how we treat our bodies greatly affects our minds and the other way around. The following section will discuss healthier choices you need to make to better control your emotions, and making these choices will improve your ability to slow down the emotional roller coaster.

Balance your sleep

Sleep is important for restoring your optimal daily functioning, and a lack of it can make you sensitive and emotionally aroused to stressful situations. Good sleep is key in your ability to cope with the emotional instability you experience in your daily life. While proper sleep helps regulate your emotions, lack of it can be detrimental to your emotional health and cause distress.

Aim to have at least eight to ten hours of sleep daily for effective emotional functioning. Getting an adequate amount of sleep helps promote improved health and mood.

Reduce caffeine and other stimulants

Many people rely on caffeine and other stimulants to keep themselves awake and energized. But do you know that caffeine and other stimulants can negatively affect your sleep and cause emotional instability? Caffeine can stay in your system for as long as 14 hours, so when you consume it in the middle of the day, that can affect your sleep later and make you feel uneasy.

Since we are all different, things may affect us differently. I want you to conduct an experiment for two weeks. Avoid taking caffeine and other stimulants during this time, and then pay attention to how you feel after the experiment. Do you feel better or worse? If you have improved sleep, that's a sign for you to reduce your caffeine intake.

Balance your nutrition

People's popular idea about balanced nutrition is that it is crucial only for optimal physical health. But do you know that eating a balanced meal also plays a crucial role in stabilizing your emotions? What you eat plays a role in hormonal balance and good mental health. To achieve emotional balance, ensure you improve your nutrition. Include a sensible proportion of proteins, carbohydrates, fats, and other beneficial nutrients in your meals. Also, stay hydrated by drinking enough fluids.

Start exercising

There are so many reasons for you to start exercising, including keeping you healthy and maintaining a healthy weight. However, it goes beyond that; exercising benefits your emotional health. It is a powerful drug without side effects (unless you have an adverse medical condition).

Engage in physical activities such as biking, walking, yoga, dancing, and Tai chi. Engaging in these exercises regularly will help improve your sleep, enhance your mood, increase your energy level, and reduce stress and feelings of depression. So, the next time you notice yourself feeling angry, stressed, and anxious, that may be a sign for you to start moving.

CHAPTER 4: MINDFUL LIVING

How often do you find yourself distracted from thinking about your present moment?

You are most likely to be distracted by thinking about everything but the present. Maybe you are working on a project, and instead of focusing on it, you are thinking about the football game you've planned with your friends for the weekend, the fight you had with your best friend, or what you will buy for your girlfriend for Valentine's Day. Perhaps, you are slightly thinking about what you are currently doing, but without your full attention. Does this sound familiar? I am guessing it does.

When you are mindful, you bring your attention back to what you are doing in the present. Being mindful is when you are working on a project, and your attention wanders to the football game you have with your friends for the weekend — you notice that your mind has wandered, so you carefully guide your attention back to the present. When your mind wanders, you notice it and do your best to bring your attention to what you are doing at that moment. This chapter will focus on the importance of mindful living and how you can use the act of mindfulness to control intense emotions and be in charge of what you feel.

Practicing Mindfulness

Mindfulness is a core DBT skill that wakes you up to life. Before you can change something, you need to wake up to it and be aware of it, and that is what mindfulness stands for. You need to be aware of your reality, your reaction, your influence over others, and what's happening around you.

When you are mindful, you are doing one thing at a time and doing it with your full attention and acceptance. You will realize that the world isn't passing you by anymore as you become more aware of your self, emotions, feelings, thoughts, and the physical sensations in your body. You will become more aware of what's going on in your surroundings and can get involved in it.

Leaving the Judgments Out

Many of us aren't aware that our words can negatively affect our emotions. When we judge, we are intensifying the emotions we experience. Think about it—have you ever been so frustrated, angry, and annoyed about something that you vent to someone about it? You may start saying things like, "Why would he say such stupid things to me?" or "That was so ridiculous of him to do that."

Think about the judgments you've made here (i.e., stupid and ridiculous). What have they done to your emotions? As you vent, does it make you feel better? The answer should be no; I don't think that approach can make you feel better. In fact, it makes you feel worse.

Now do you understand the impact of judging your emotions? It keeps you on a roller coaster of emotions and increases emotional pain. Not sure of this? Okay, next time you have an argument with your friend or something happens with your parents, try venting to someone about it. Retell the story and use those judgments the way you normally would. However, this time, really notice yourself as you vent. Be aware of what happens to your emotions and your internal experience. Are they the same throughout the process of telling the story? Is there a decrease or an increase? Do you feel calm and relaxed, or do you feel tense? Does your voice remain calm as you tell the story, or do you notice the volume of your voice changing as you speak? After you've finished venting, do you feel better, worse, or the same?

Research has revealed that venting out will only make you relive the experience, which means those painful emotions will increase as you tell the story, and this can make you feel worse rather than better.

Below are some mindfulness exercises that can help you reduce your physical and emotional pain, make you feel relaxed and calm, increase positive emotions (self-control, memory, and concentration), and ultimately help you find balance.

Exercise: Mindful Listening

This exercise aims to enhance your hearing ability in a non-judgmental way and train your mind to not sway as a result of misconceptions and past experiences. You may not be aware of it, but what you feel right now may be influenced by your past experiences. For example, you dislike a particular song because it reminds you of a breakup that ended badly, so you tend to be sad any time you hear the song. The idea of this exercise is to experience the trigger from a neutral point. In this case, we'll use a song; listen to a song with the presence of your awareness and without any preconception.

Choose a song you've never listened to before. You can just go online or use the radio to choose a song that catches your ear.

- Put on your headphones and close your eyes.
- Before listening to the song, ensure you don't get drawn into judging the music by its title, genre, or artist. Ignore any of these labels and free yourself by getting lost in the song's rhythm and sound.
- Explore all aspects of the track without any reservations. You may not like the music at first but try to let go of the dislike and allow yourself to be fully aware as you enter into the track, dancing among the waves of the song.

- Listen to every dynamic of every instrument used in the song. In your mind, separate each sound and analyze them one after the other.
- Home in on the vocals, including the tone of the voice, sound, and range. Separate the voices if there is more than one.

The aim of this exercise is for you to listen with intention and become fully entwined in the composition of the song without any form of judgment. You don't need to think, just hear.

Exercise: Mindful Eating

Mindful eating involves paying attention to the food you are about to eat, noticing how it feels in your hands, focusing on its weight, texture, and color, and bringing about an awareness of its smell. This also involves chewing your food slowly, with full concentration. You should also notice the texture and taste against your tongue. This exercise will help you discover new experiences with foods.

Below is an assessment of your mindful eating skills. This assessment will help you identify the skills you need to improve and those you are already doing well with.

Tick (✔) the option that applies to you best.

I stop eating when I am full

At all times:
Most times:
Occasionally:
Sometimes:
Almost never:

I pick or graze on food

At all times:
Most times:
Occasionally:
Sometimes:
Almost never:

I eat when I am hungry, not when I am emotional

At all times:

Most times:

Occasionally:

Sometimes:

Almost never:

I am nonjudgmental of my body when I accidentally overeat

At all times:

Most times:

Occasionally:

Sometimes:

Almost never:

I taste every bite of food properly before reaching for the next

At all times:

Most times:

Occasionally:

Sometimes:

Almost never:

I think about the nourishment the food gives my body when I eat

> *At all times:*
>
> *Most times:*
>
> *Occasionally:*
>
> *Sometimes:*
>
> *Almost never:*

I don't do any other thing when I eat; I just eat

> *At all times:*
>
> *Most times:*
>
> *Occasionally:*
>
> *Sometimes:*
>
> *Almost never:*

I eat slowly and chew every bite

> *At all times:*
>
> *Most times:*
>
> *Occasionally:*
>
> *Sometimes:*
>
> *Almost never:*

I don't have to eat everything on my plate; I can stop eating when I am full

> *At all times:*
>
> *Most times:*
>
> *Occasionally:*
>
> *Sometimes:*
>
> *Almost never:*

I do realize when I zone out when eating and carefully guide my focus to the food

> *At all times:*
>
> *Most times:*
>
> *Occasionally:*
>
> *Sometimes:*
>
> *Almost never:*

What are your mindful eating goals?

(Example: slowing down when eating, being more present, or stopping when full).

- _____

- _____

- _____

Exercise: Observe-a-Leaf Mindfulness

This very simple mindfulness exercise requires just your attention and a leaf. To do this:

- Pick a leaf and hold it in your hand.
- Focus on the leaf for five minutes, giving it your full attention.
- Notice the shape, color, patterns, and texture of the leaf.

This simple exercise will bring your awareness to the present and connect your thoughts with your present experience.

Exercise: Mindfulness Breathing

Many mindfulness breathing exercises can help you. So, I will be explaining some of those that are easy to practice.

Square Breathing:

- Breath in and hold your breath for four seconds.
- Breath out for four seconds.
- Repeat the process four times, and that's it!

Deep Breathing:

- Breath in through your nose.
- Breath out through your mouth.
- Quiet your mind and increase your focus by saying "in" when you breathe in and "out" when you breathe out.

Breathing Colors:

- Choose two colors (one for breathing in and one for breathing out).
- Picture a color for the breath-in and the other for the breath-out.
- Choose the colors you want and for the reasons you want them.
- Now, close your eyes and pair the colors with your breaths.

Belly Breathing:

- Lie down on the floor or bed, or just sit upright in a chair.
- Place your hands on your belly.
- Slowly breathe in and watch how your belly is expanding.

When you breathe this way, you promote deep breathing, which aids the transportation of oxygen into your system. You need more oxygen for relaxation and thinking clearly.

3-Step Mindfulness Worksheet

This worksheet is designed to help you practice mindfulness in three steps and bring your awareness to the present.

1. Step Away from Autopilot

In the first step, you will be bringing your awareness to what you are thinking, doing, and sensing at the moment. You will need to pause, stay in a comfortable position, be relaxed, and breathe.

What do you feel right now? What are the thoughts coming up in your mind?

Once you've identified them, give them your attention and notice them as natural experiences. Allow them to pass; slowly adjust to your current state and who you are.

2. Be Aware of Your Breath

Your goal at the moment is to be aware of your breath.

As you breathe in and out, how does your body move? Is your chest rising as you let air in and falling as you let the air out?

Once you know the pattern of your breath, anchor yourself to the present moment with what you've realized and take six breaths.

3. *Expand Your Awareness Outwardly*

In the last stage, you should allow your awareness to spread outwardly. It should start with your body and with your surroundings.

What are those physical sensations you are experiencing? Take note of any aches, feelings of lightness, or tightness, and let them go.

Now expand your awareness outwardly. Focus your attention on what's in front of you.

What shapes, colors, and textures can you notice?

Notice and be present in the awareness of those things.

Exercise: Mindful Immersion (Attention Workout)

This exercise aims to help you cultivate contentment with the moment and escape the constant hardship you get caught up in daily. It encourages you to engage in your regular routine and fully experience it, rather than anxiously wanting to get done with it to enable you to start something else.

The exercise encourages creativity so you can discover new experiences while doing a certain task. Whether you are cleaning your house or doing any other task, the aim is to pay attention to every little detail and notice every aspect of the task and your actions. For example, when sweeping the floor, you should feel and become the motion involved. You could sense your muscles as you scrub the dishes or have an efficient way of wiping a window clean.

Now, think of those routines you do daily. It can be taking a shower, washing, gardening, folding clothes, walking, brushing your teeth, and eating.

Write down any of the routines and where you want to do them.

It's time to write where your attention is focused. Is it self-focused attention (focused on your thoughts, feelings, emotions, and symptoms) or task-focused emotion (focused on the task)?

- Start doing the task without intentionally bringing your attention to it.
- Whenever you notice that your attention is wandering away from the task, carefully move your attention back to it without any form of judgment. Focus on:

Taste: What flavors do you notice? How many of them? Are they constant, or do they change during the task?

Sight: What are the things you can notice about the task? How does the task look? What catches your attention? Do you notice light, colors, and shadows?

Smell: What smell do you notice most? How many smells can you notice? Is the smell constant, or does it change during the task?

Touch: What task do you engage in? What does doing it feel like? What is the texture like? Is it rough or smooth? What part of your body are you using for the task?

Hearing: What sounds can you notice? What sounds can you link to the task?

After completing this task, where did you notice your attention focused during the task?

What have you learned from the task, and what's your conclusion about the task?

You don't need to write down your answers to every question above if you choose not to. I've provided them to remind you that you need awareness of all your sense organs during every task. You can use the senses to shift your awareness back to the task when it wanders.

Finally, you can practice the act of mindfulness when in any difficult situation. In fact, you can practice it any time. Mindfulness doesn't advocate perfection; it's just about practicing how to improve your awareness of things. As you practice mindfulness, be compassionate with yourself. Life won't always be rosy. There are stressful times too, but you will feel better despite the difficulties when you use compassion and mindfulness.

CHAPTER 5: MANAGING ANXIETY, ANGER, TRAUMA, AND PTSD WITH DBT

Even though DBT is popular for treating borderline personality disorder (BPD), it has a simple foundation. The concept is used for fostering change and acceptance. It allows people with other mental health conditions, such as anxiety, depression, anger, trauma, and PTSD, to accept the present, knowing that their future must be changed.

Managing Anxiety and Depression with DBT

One in every five Americans has a form of anxiety or an anxiety disorder. However, the good news is that research has revealed that DBT is very effective in helping anxious people manage their anxiety and live better lives.

With DBT, you can either work independently or with a therapist to find and resolve the contradictions between your present and your desired state of being. You will get a treatment plan that encourages positive behavioral changes.

The following are DBT techniques you can use to manage anxiety.

One-mindedness

This is a skill that encourages being in the moment. People often live in their present life thinking and worrying about their past or future. This can trigger anxiety as you get yourself stuck in thinking about what you've done wrong or what you think you will do wrong.

Being in the present moment will prepare you to better handle future problems and not worry about the past. When you worry constantly, it can be crippling — damaging your psyche to the extent that it becomes difficult to recognize effective actions or follow through with them.

When you engage fully in the present, you can easily deal with future issues that may arise. You also get to keep anxiety at bay because you will be fostering fewer worries about the past and so have a more mentally-grounded perspective to deal with future problems.

Exercise: Mindfulness of your current thoughts

Observe your thoughts:

- Notice as the waves come and go.
- Don't suppress, analyze, or judge your thoughts.
- Acknowledge the presence of your thoughts.
- Don't keep your thoughts around.
- Step away and observe your thoughts as they come in and escape your mind.

Have a curious mind:

- Ask yourself where your thoughts are coming from.
- Acknowledge that each thought that comes to your mind also goes out.
- Observe your thoughts without evaluating them.

Know that you aren't your thoughts:

- Don't act on your thoughts.
- Remember the times when you had different thoughts.
- Acknowledge that a catastrophic thought is from an emotional mind.
- Remember how you think when you don't feel pain and suffering.

Don't suppress your thoughts:

- Figure out the sensations your thoughts are trying to block off.
- Focus on the sensations and return to the thoughts after a moment.
- Step away by allowing your thoughts to come and go while observing your breath.
- Start playing with your thoughts by repeating them out loud as fast as you can.
- Love your thoughts.

Self-Soothing

This is the act of calming your emotional roller coaster by grounding yourself using your five senses. Most times, anxious people can easily get stuck in the emotional turmoil of their minds. You can escape your mind and enter the physical world again with the self-soothing technique. Instead of worrying and ruminating, DBT encourages you to gain relief through your senses.

Exercise: Self-soothing with the senses

In the worksheet below, write down pleasurable ways to soothe yourself. Write the fun things you would like to do when experiencing a difficult day.

Senses	Activities
Taste	Example: Chew gum or drink a cup of tea. ● _____ ● _____
Sight	Example: Watch my favorite movie or sit outside and bask in nature. ● _____ ● _____

Sound	Example: Listen to my favorite song or positive affirmations. • _____ • _____
Smell	Example: Light up a scented candle or diffuse essential oils • _____ • _____
Touch	Example: Take a warm bath or get a massage • _____ • _____

Radical Acceptance

This technique requires you to accept the world exactly the way it is at the moment. I know that may sound easy, but it isn't. How easy is it to accept a painful breakup, the death of a loved one, or failing an exam?

The scope behind radical acceptance isn't to turn your back on the painful experiences but to accept that they happened; they are real and true. Therefore, your mental effort should be focused on making peace with an experience or changing it.

Exercise: Improving the moment

When faced with anxiety, you should improve the moment by:

- **Imagining** yourself dealing with the problem successfully
- Finding **meaning** in the difficult situation
- **Praying** to a higher power asking for strength to tolerate the pain a little longer
- **Relaxing**
- Focusing on **one thing** at a time
- **Vacationing** in your mind
- **Encouraging** yourself

So how can you apply this?

Imagining	Visualize a secret room within yourself or a relaxing scene. Daydream about your favorite place or memory.

Meaning	Recall the important things in your life. What can you learn from the tough times you've experienced? Have you survived a similar situation before?
Praying	Meditate, pray, or ponder about it. Use your spirituality.
Relaxing	Use calming techniques such as deep breathing. Don't prevent the event; allow it to unfold.
Being in the moment	Be aware of what you are doing in the moment and focus on one thing at a time.
Vacationing	Take a break.
Encouraging	Use positive affirmations or make helpful statements about yourself and others.

Exercise: Pros and cons list

This exercise entails making a list of the pros and cons of a situation to help you decide if you should act on the anxiety-based urge or go with a healthier decision.

	Pros	Cons
Coping	• No argument • No fight • Gaining others' trust • Having more privileges • Increased self-esteem • Maintain relationship	• You don't get to argue or fight • You fail to make your point • There's no instant gratification • Others won't fear you
Not Coping	• You will be left alone • Hurting someone • Instant gratification • Feeling powerful	• Low self-worth • Lost self-esteem • Lost respect • Lost motivation for getting treated • Rebellion against using skills

Now, ask yourself which of the pros and cons listed above are short-term (one day) and which are long-term (more than one day). If you've identified them, ask your wise mind if you would rather experience a good day or a good life. Then make a mindful choice of action.

Making sensible decisions when you're anxious can be difficult. Using the pros and cons list can help individuals decide if they should act on an anxiety-based urge or develop a healthier decision.

Exercise: TIPP

TIPP is an acronym that stands for temperature, intense exercise, paced breathing, and paired muscle relaxation.

You can practice TIPP when you experience anxiety by:

- Cooling your body **temperature** (this calms you emotionally too)
- Practicing an **intense exercise** to match your intense emotions
- **Pacing** your breathing
- Engaging in **paired muscle relaxation**

The exercises I've shared can help you prepare for intense emotions and cope with distressing feelings in a better way.

Managing Anger with DBT

If you experience anger that turns into rage, say things in the heat of the moment and eventually regret it, or are looking for coping strategies to help you cope with your anger, then this section is for you.

Anger can be damaging to the extent that it affects what you do or say before you can even recognize the emotion. When you express anger all the time, you may get so used to the emotion that you don't notice when it's there. The first step to take when managing anger is identifying those warning signs that tell you how you feel.

When you are angry, how do you react? Some warning signs may show themselves when you feel a little irritated, while others show up when you are very angry. Tick (✓) the warning signs that apply to you in the following table.

Warning signs

Face turns red

Mind goes blank

Insult the person

Scream or yell

Throw things

Argue

Hand and body shake

Punch walls

Start sweating

Cry

Become aggressive

Headaches

Pace around

Feel hot inside

The next exercise offers steps you can take to overcome the anger.

Know your anger sign	Use the list of warning signs above to know your anger sign.
Take a time-out	Leave the situation that's making you angry, even if temporarily. Take a few minutes to calm down.

Engage in deep breathing	Practice deep breathing by counting your breaths. Inhale and count four seconds; exhale and count four seconds.
Exercise	Exercise triggers chemicals to be released in your brain to create a sense of happiness and relaxation.
Express your anger	Express your frustration after calming down. Be assertive and not aggressive.
Know the consequences of your anger	What can be the result of your anger-fueled actions? Will throwing things convince the person that you are right? Will you be happy with your actions?
Visualize a better outcome	Imagine having a relaxed experience. What can you see, hear, smell, taste, and touch? Spend a few minutes imagining being in your ideal environment.

Managing Trauma and PTSD with DBT

Whether you are suffering from panic attacks, un-relenting worries, or a phobia due to trauma and PTSD, you don't need to continue living this way.

With DBT, you don't need to burden your mind with worries or live in fear. DBT encourages people living with trauma to face their fears rather than avoid them. Exposing yourself to fearful thoughts and situations will eventually reduce the pain that comes with them.

But how can you do this, especially when it's very uncomfortable? The following exercises will help you manage your feelings and live a better life.

Exercise: Assess your limitations

This exercise aims to assess your limitation of trauma-provoking thoughts and situations. The response you give will encourage you to break free from the shackles of your past.

What thoughts or situations have prevented you from pursuing your goals and living your best life?

How would you act differently if you overcame this experience and focused on what's important?

What are your thoughts and feelings when faced with the experience?

What steps can you take to overcome the trauma?

List five things you can do to face trauma-based thoughts.

After accomplishing the steps listed, how can you use them to manage trauma in the future?

Exercise: Work through the trauma and live your best life

This exercise entails doing certain activities to help you work through your trauma, stop being a hostage of your thoughts, and start living your best life.

Sit with your fear: When the thoughts come, don't avoid them. Just sit with them for three minutes. Remind yourself that being scared is natural, and you will eventually be in charge of your thoughts. After three minutes, start doing an activity you enjoy, such as singing, dancing, or painting.

Encourage yourself: When a difficult and painful thought comes, tell yourself that you won't allow fear to limit you or prevent you from achieving your goals. Remind yourself of how strong you are and that you shouldn't be stopped and attacked by your thoughts.

Start exercising: Start engaging in exercise to help you refocus your mind toward more important things. Go for a walk, do yoga, or start dancing. This will also boost the confidence you need to face any situation.

Write a gratitude list: Your gratitude list should contain the things that make you grateful. When you feel down and in a bad place, look at the list and recall the things you have that you're thankful for. This will make you feel better.

Use humor to deflate your worries: Use humor to reduce your fears and worries when discomforting thoughts appear. For example, when thinking of the heartbreak you experienced and how you were jilted, you can say to yourself, *"What's the worst-case scenario? He probably wasn't the one for me, and I know I will love again."* Or, when you lose a loved one, you can say, *"Death is a natural phenomenon that will happen to us all. Maybe not now, but eventually."*

CHAPTER 6: THE ROAD TO POSITIVE EMOTIONS (IMPROVING YOUR MOOD)

From the beginning of this book, we've been discussing skills that can help you manage painful and discomforting emotions and prevent you from experiencing emotional pain. I believe you've been practicing these skills and have started seeing results, no matter how small. Meanwhile, there is an important aspect we need to discuss, and that is your mood. Unfortunately, despite the skills you've learned and practiced, your mood will likely not improve unless you focus on seeking to improve it.

You probably think this is another process that requires hard work, and you aren't sure if you are up for that. But doesn't feeling better require hard work? If you regularly feel anxious, depressed, nervous, angry, irritated, annoyed, and trauma-tized, then you need to put in the work to improve your mood and slow down the emotional roller-coaster you've been riding. This is what this final chapter will focus on—smoothing out the roller-coaster ride by improving your mood.

First, we'll start with having a goal and working toward it before other steps can follow.

Work Toward a Goal

If you want to improve your mood and your life in general, goal setting is important. You are head-ing toward failure if you live a life without goals. Therefore, it is important to set goals that will en-courage accountability.

Goal-setting can help you face emotional and be-havioral challenges, improve your savings habits, score better grades in school, and build better re-lationships. It is your roadmap to success when trying to overcome challenges and live a better life.

To help you set effective goals, we'll be discussing the SMART rule, which stands for making your goals Specific, Measurable, Achievable, Realistic, and Time-bound.

Set SMART Goals

There are different approaches to executing your plans, and an effective one is the SMART way. Setting SMART goals will give you a better idea of your objectives and encourage you to achieve them.

Exercise: Making your goals SMART

Write your response in the box below.

SPECIFIC

What would you like to achieve? Ensure your goal is specific and broken down into smaller steps.

MEASURABLE

Write how you can make your goals measurable. How would you know when your aims have been achieved? What difference do you expect? What will you be doing seldom and doing regularly?

ACHIEVABLE

What are the achievable goals you can set to avoid failure? You can set smaller goals and celebrate when you achieve a milestone.

REALISTIC

What resources do you have at your disposal? Are they enough to achieve your goals? Do you need extra resources? If you do, do you have access to them or not? What challenges do you experience when accessing them? What are the steps you need to take to remove these challenges?

TIME-BOUND

What is the reasonable timeline you can set for achieving your goals? The timeline can be a day, a week, a month, a year, or more. Break down the goals and note a timeline for each of the steps.

What changes can you effect to improve your mood and your life generally? Write them down below.

1. Changes with family:

_____

2. Changes at school:

_____

3. Changes with friends:

_____

4. Changes in extra-curriculum activities (music, sports, and work):

_____

What would you like to focus on first?

_____

_____

_____

What are your possible obstacles?

What can you do to overcome these obstacles?

When do you want to make these changes?

If you aren't sure that the SMART rule for goal setting will be helpful, or if you can't seem to set meaningful goals by using it, you can switch your plan and use another technique for goal setting.

Use a technique that has a solid plan and will give results.

If you want to see results with SMART goal setting, you will need to be patient with the process. Though it may take time, especially with long-term goals. I encourage you to hang in there and be patient with the process.

In your planning, don't try to comply with "all or nothing" rules because you have a variety of goals, and you can't achieve all of them at once. Not achieving them at the same time doesn't mean you are a failure. Celebrate the little ones you've achieved and prepare for the bigger ones. When you fail to achieve a goal, take your time to have a better plan in place to prevent failure the next time you attempt it.

Building Mastery

While goal setting is important, you need to engage in pleasurable activities to strike a balance and make you feel fulfilled. The DBT skill of building mastery encourages you to engage in activities that will make you feel productive and proud of yourself for achieving something. The list for building mastery mustn't be the same as that of anyone else; it's different for everyone. While it may be auditioning for the school play for one person, it could be making it to school on time for another. What really matters is that the activity should give you a pleasant and positive feeling about yourself.

Think about what you are doing in your life that gives you a positive and pleasurable feeling. What else can you do to make sure you have this sense of fulfillment regularly?

Engaging in Pleasurable Activities

It's advisable to engage in different activities to boost your mood and achieve mental wellness. According to studies, exercises can help produce endorphins in your body. Endorphins are feel-good hormones that boost your mood and make you happy and energized. Examples of such exercises include breathing practices, yoga, meditation, visualization, and other fun activities. Engaging in any exercise regularly is beneficial to your health and state of mind.

The following are activities you can engage in:

Focused Hobbies

This involves taking some time off to read articles, paint, walk, watch a movie, learn a musical instrument, or go shopping. Get yourself a hobby that will take your thoughts off your usual routine. The idea is to refresh and re-energize your mind. If you need to change your environment to get it done, don't hesitate to do that.

Visualization

Imagine yourself in a calm and relaxed place. This can be lying on a beach, sitting on top of a mountain, or lounging under a tree. While you are in this calm state, what can you see? What can you taste? What can you feel? What can you smell? What can you hear? What are your thoughts? Your discovery should make you feel relaxed and able to enjoy the moment.

Deep Breathing

We've discussed practicing deep breathing in Chapters 4 and 5, so you should be familiar with it already. Deep breathing entails focusing your attention on your breath for a few minutes. Inhale through your nose and count to four, hold your breath for four seconds, exhale through your mouth, and count for another four seconds.

Improve Your Relationships

As you survive the emotional roller coaster and learn skills that will help you manage your emotions more beneficially, it's pertinent to improve your relationship with your friends, family, teacher, coaches, and love interests. This can positively affect your mood and influence how well you manage your emotions.

We are social creatures that need people around us. When you have healthy and satisfying relationships, you can be more emotionally resilient. The people around you greatly influence your feelings, so it's important to continually improve the bond you have with them.

A major component of DBT is interpersonal effectiveness, or improving your relationship with others. Therefore, the following techniques aim to help you accomplish that.

GIVE Skills

The GIVE skills entail:

- Be **gentle.** Be nice and respectful and avoid any form of physical and verbal attacks. Don't engage in gestures that are insulting and threatening. For example, don't roll your eyes, clench your fists, smirk, or hiss.

- Be **interested**. Even when you aren't absorbed in what the other person is saying, act interested by maintaining eye contact and giving listening ears. Don't interrupt or talk over them.

- **Validate** them. When you validate, you show that you understand their point of view and why they do what they do.

- Use an **easy manner.** Remember to use easy manners such as humor and smiling.

FAST Skills

These skills will help you preserve your self-respect when interacting with others. To do this:

- Be **fair** to yourself and others. Appreciate your worth and needs.

- Don't over-**apologize**. This doesn't mean you shouldn't apologize when you are at fault. It means you shouldn't apologize for having a different opinion or asking for what you need.

- **Stick** to your values. Communicate what you believe in clearly, and don't be afraid to stand up for your opinion when it comes to your values.

- Be **truthful** and don't lie. When you lie to get what you want, you will compromise your relationship with others and lose self-respect.

DEAR MAN

This is an interpersonal skill that you can use to ask for what you want, respectfully and effectively, thereby building and maintaining wholesome relationships with others, regardless of whether or not you get what you asked for.

To do this:

- **Describe** the situation simply. If you want to go shopping with your friend, you can describe the situation in a straightforward way by saying, "My friends are going to the mall to shop for new clothes this weekend."

- **Express** what you would like to do. For example, "I would like to go shopping with them."

- **Assert** respectfully and not aggressively why it is important to you. For example, "I haven't spent time with my friends since track season started, so it would mean a lot if I could go with them this weekend."

- **Reinforce** when you get what you asked for. For example, "I promise to do all my homework before I leave for shopping."

- **Mindfully** stay in the moment. Don't worry about your past or future; just be in the moment. For example, don't worry about what your friends will say if you cancel going out.

- **Appear** confident. Don't be afraid to ask your friends to give you more time to focus on your homework instead, if that's what you need. Approach the situation confidently.

- **Negotiate** if it looks like you won't get your desired result. Many teenagers aren't used to asking for something; they would rather make demands and ask in uncertain ways that seem confusing. Or they would rather not ask at all and just do what they want. So, it's important to be flexible and find a happy middle ground for both yourself and the other person.

Interpersonal effectiveness skills aren't just for helping those struggling with BPD; it is helpful for anyone who wants to strengthen the relationships they have with the people around them.

FINAL WORDS

Well done! You've finally reached the end of this book, and I must commend you for staying with me all the way. It's been an exciting experience, walking through this journey with you, and I believe you've learned the invaluable skills of DBT. These skills will help you make positive changes in your life and achieve mental wellness.

I believe that you now know:

- What DBT entails and how you can utilize its skills
- How to identify the times when you have unhealthy thoughts and the exercises you can use to focus on the moment instead of acting on those thoughts
- Important strategies you can use to manage anxiety, anger, trauma, and PTSD

- How to reevaluate your life and set goals for the next stage of your life
- How to improve your mood by engaging in pleasurable activities
- How to build better relationships

You might encounter obstacles along the way as you strive to live a healthier and better life. However, I trust you won't give up and let the hard work you've invested in this journey go to waste. Keep moving forward, and you will get your reward shortly.

I've shared effective skills, techniques, and exercises to improve your mental health. As with any form of therapy, DBT requires work on your part. So I encourage you not to give up; keep practicing what you've learned in this book, and in no time, you will get your desired results.

FREE BONUS

Overcome Anxiety Book

How To Stop The Cycle Of Anxiety, Worry & Fear So You Can Regain Control Of Your Life Forever

Scan The Code To Get This FREE Book.

(Your mobile camera has a built-in scanner.)

DOWNLOADABLE WORKSHEETS

Please go to the below URL to download all worksheets (in pdf format) given in the book.

Https://TheMentorBucket.com/dbt_ws.pdf

MORE RECOMMENDED BOOKS

Please go to the below URL and check our recommended books.

Https://TheMentorBucket.Com/resources

CPSIA information can be obtained
at www.ICGtesting.com
Printed in the USA
BVHW040912030722
641203BV00002BA/48

9 781955 906036